Copyright Notice

First Printing, 2012

ISBN-13: 978-1475194968

ISBN-10: 147519496X

Printed in the United States of America

Table of Contents

Introduction

Thank you for picking up your copy of Tired of Feeling Tired.

Fatigue, tiredness, exhaustion, lethargy or whatever name you have for it is a major problem and is one of the main reasons people go to visit the doctor.

My hope is that by the time you've finished reading this book you'll have a better understanding of what is causing you to feel fatigued and that you'll have a good solid list of preventative measures you can take to reverse this plight on your life.

So who am I and what makes me qualified to write a book on this topic? Well my name is James Driver and I'm in my mid 40's. I am a qualified personal trainer and my degree is in Sport Science.

I don't remember having problems with feeling tired while I was a child, but I certainly started noticing its onset around high school, probably at the age of 13. Outwardly I was a completely healthy looking child and grew up into an outwardly healthy looking young man. However, inside I was always feeling very tired and even exhausted.

This carried on through university and into my working life. I changed jobs, the years ticked by and I was still feeling tired throughout large portions of the day. This highly affected my productivity, my relationships and my entire life. Feeling tired in an evening and on the weekend would stop me from going out and having fun like everybody else.

So when I reached my mid 30's I decided to start researching this, almost to the extent of it becoming an obsession. I never intended to write a book about how to overcome being tired all the time, but I was able to help myself become a fully energized member of the community once again.

I soon noticed that my personal training clients were asking me about fatigue en masse. When I started giving advice to others around me, my clients and friends, then later on an internet forum, I decided to write this book to help many others who were having their life blighted by some mystery, hidden burden that was destroying their lives in silence, most often without being diagnosed.

So admittedly I don't have any formal medical qualifications. So if you're after medical mumbo jumbo then you're reading the wrong book. All I can offer you in Tired of Feeling Tired is my own perspective of how I cured my tiredness and how I helped cure other people's tiredness, fatigue or whatever you would like to call it.

In any case, as many of us will know the medical world has failed to agree on a name for this condition, they have failed to find a way of diagnosing it with any consistency and they have certainly failed to find a cure. So not having a medical background myself, I'll take as a badge of honour.

I am based in the UK, a tiring country, so if you're not based in England, you'll have to excuse my Englishisms.

I am intending this book to be fairly light and as simple as possible. Many of the books I've read on this subject are extremely heavy on the medical language and targeted at people with PhD's. Since I'm an ordinary guy myself, I'm targeting this book at ordinary men and women who reach lunch hour and feel like they need a long sleep, who get home after work and collapse on the bed, who fail to get up in the morning due to exhaustion, who can't muster the energy to go to a bar with friends for a drink. This book is not for university professors, it's for the guy or girl who really needs it.

This book is going to be split into a few different sections. Firstly, I'm going to briefly mention a few of the conditions you may possibly have which could be causing your fatigue. I will explain the subtle differences between them so that hopefully you along with a doctor will be able to rule them out.

Then we'll talk about the effects of fatigue on people's lives, which will be very brief.

After that, we'll discuss the causes of fatigue, something that is essential you understand so you know how to better combat it. In the same section we'll also talk about how you can combat the causes of fatigue.

Finally we'll take a look at a few extra preventative measures and cures for finally defeating fatigue in order to give you maximum energy for the rest of your life.

I hope we succeed in this together!

Section 1

The Many Forms of Fatigue

Below are some of the known medical conditions and health problems which are known to cause fatigue.

If you suffer from fatigue then it's a possibility you suffer from one of the following conditions. However, it's known that one in four people suffers from general fatigue without suffering from a known medical condition.

The best course of action for yourself would be to rule out each of the below conditions with a doctor. Once a known medical condition has been ruled out, then you probably are one of the one in four. This book will be of great help to you in that case!

The reason there is little agreement within the medical community regarding the many conditions which cause fatigue is that symptoms often overlap. In addition, fatigue may actually be one of many symptoms you're experiencing due to the condition or illness you're suffering from. I also name some common conditions where fatigue is just one symptom below.

Chronic Fatigue Syndrome (CFS) / Myalgic Encephalomyelitis (ME)

CFS is probably the most common term used by the medical profession when talking about fatigue. There are no ways of diagnosing it!

As well as tiredness, other symptoms often include; muscle and joint pain as well as headaches. It is estimated 1 million people in America have CFS and over a quarter of a million in the UK, mainly effecting females.

ME in particular has widely been given the name in the media as the "lazy disease!" Understanding of the condition is practically non-existent. Many sufferers prefer the term ME to CFS since it is believed the term Chronic Fatigue Syndrome trivialises the condition, stops it from being seen as a genuine medical condition and prevents research from taking place. The two terms are often used interchangeably even though the medical definition of ME is "inflammation of the brain and spinal cord with muscle pain." I hope I've made my point in that there is much still to be known about this condition, especially considering they use CFS interchangeably with ME.

The definition of CFS according to the Centres for Disease Control and Prevention in America is that you have to fulfil these two criteria:

1. A new onset (not lifelong) of unexplained, persistent fatigue unrelated to exertion and not

substantially relieved by rest, that causes a significant reduction in previous activity levels.

2. In addition, you must suffer from at least four or perhaps more of the following symptoms; impaired memory or concentration, post exertional malaise, unrefreshing sleep, muscle pain, joint pain, headaches, sore throat and tender lymph nodes.

Post Viral Fatigue Syndrome (PVFS)

PVFS has almost identical symptoms to CFS with the addition of loss of appetite. As the name suggests PVFS would involve long bouts of fatigue following a viral infection, often lasting for months or years, either sporadically or constantly.

Research into risk factors of PVFS has been contradictory at best. Some studies have shown the severity of the viral infection to be a risk factor for PVFS [1] while other studies have sited genetic, demographic and psychological reasons for PVFS [2].

Once again there are huge disagreements within the medical community with regards to PVFS.

Fibromyalgia

Once again fatigue is just one of the symptoms of fibromyalgia! In fact, if you have fibromyalgia, fatigue will be the least of your worries. You'll also have as symptoms; widespread pain especially when pressure is applied to your joints, muscle pain, nerve pain, palpitations, bowel and bladder abnormalities as well as difficulty swallowing, numbing and tingling. Psychologically you'll suffer from depression and anxiety to an extent.

Fibromyalgia is actually quite common affecting around 3% of the population in western countries; 90% being in women.

Although Fibromyalgia can now be diagnosed, there is no known cure!

I doubt that many people I've spoken to over the years were suffering from fibromyalgia as sufferers are more likely to be receiving treatment for their other symptoms as a priority over their fatigue.

Anaemia

Even though if you have anaemia you're quite likely to already know about it, I've included this section to cover all bases.

So what is anaemia and how does it cause fatigue? Simply, anaemia is where there is a decrease in red blood cells or in the haemoglobin molecules which carry oxygen in the blood to your organs. A decrease in the ability of haemoglobin to successfully carry oxygen around your body can also be classed as a type of anaemia.

Haemoglobin is incredibly important in the functioning of our bodies. If it cannot function properly then we will feel fatigued.

The main cause of anaemia is iron deficiency in the body. Iron is a valuable component of haemoglobin. Major blood loss can also cause anaemia.

Anaemia is most commonly found in young women due to their menstrual cycles, the monthly loss of blood can cause fatigue, however the small loss of blood can easily be coped with by most people. That being said, if you do suffer from anaemia then this small loss of blood can exacerbate the symptoms of fatigue.

Anaemia brought on from an accident is the main reason we suffer dizziness, fatigue and light headedness due to heavy bleeding.

Vegetarians are also at risk from anaemia due to a lack of vitamin B12 in their diets that is found in fish, meat and eggs.

The main symptoms of anaemia are fatigue, heart palpitations, looking pale and hair loss. It affects over three million Americans.

Doctors can diagnose anaemia by taking a blood sample and analysing the quantity of red blood cells and haemoglobin in the sample. It is all very easy to carry out, it takes only a few minutes and is in fact done on a machine these days. Depending on which type of test you take, results can be given within a few minutes or an hour.

So how can anaemia be treated?

Well that will be up to your doctor and depending on the severity and kind of anaemia the patient has.

Doctors will typically first correct the underlying cause, the blood loss which the patient may be suffering from.

The patient will be advised to eat foods high in iron such as meat particularly liver, shellfish and eggs.

Iron supplements are also common as well as injections or supplements of vitamin B12.

Thyroid Disease

There are many more Americans that suffer from some kind of thyroid abnormality than suffer from diabetes.

There are different kinds of thyroid problems and they effect both men and women of all ages.

Thyroid problems can cause fatigue as well as a long list of other problems for the sufferer.

The thyroid gland, an under appreciated organ is located in the neck and is responsible for producing thyroid hormones, which serve to regulate metabolism as well as a few other things in the body.

The thyroid gland is regulated by the pituitary and hypothalamus which are located in the brain. If a malfunction occurs between these three organs then an excessive amount of thyroid hormone can be produced which results in hyperthyroidism. Any malfunction can also cause a reduction in thyroid hormone being produced which causes hypothyroidism. These are two of the different thyroid diseases which can occur and they can both lead to fatigue.

Hypothyroidism

Having an underactive thyroid can result in hypothyroidism, where you're producing too little thyroid hormone. Studies [3] have shown around 8% of people in the UK suffers from Hypothyroidism to some degree and it has even been noticed in infants. The following are some of the symptoms which can vary depending on your deficiency; fatigue, brain fog, constipation, feeling cold, fluid retention, dry skin, depression and stiff muscles and joints.

Hyperthyroidism

Having an overactive thyroid can result in hyperthyroidism, where you're producing too much thyroid hormone. The following symptoms of producing too much thyroid hormone are due to the increase in the speed of metabolism; fatigue, heat intolerance, excessive sweating, nervousness, agitation, increased bowel movements, weight loss, rapid heart rate and decreased concentration. In women hypothyroidism can affect pregnancy and fertility rates due to the increased need for thyroid hormones.

Diagnosing Thyroid Disease

Diagnosis can be carried out in a number of ways; blood tests, imaging to see the size of the thyroid gland, or a biopsy.

Treatment

Treatment for hypothyroidism involves taking thyroid hormone replacements to replace what the thyroid gland is not producing on its own.

Likewise for hyperthyroidism, the doctor can prescribe you medication that reduces the amount of hormone the gland produces.

However, fatigue is not one of the treatable symptoms. If you're diagnosed with hypothyroidism then many of your symptoms can be managed, however you'll also benefit greatly from the fatigue combatting measures in this book.

Copper Toxicity Syndrome (CTS) / Copper Imbalance

This is a funny one really because one of the symptoms of CTS is hyperactivity. Having excess copper in the body can have similar effects as having increased levels of caffeine. Clearly this is the opposite of fatigue!

Yet again however, there is a long list of symptoms which include two of the above; Fibromyalgia and Hypothyroidism. This has led one world renowned researcher [4] and scientist to hypothesize that CTS is a cause of fatigue.

Having high copper levels in your blood is something that is becoming very common these days and has a long list of alarming symptoms; acne, hair loss, anaemia, anxiety, arthritis, depression, infertility, migraines, PMS, chronic infections, insomnia, nerve pain, hypertension and schizophrenia.

The reason there are contradictory conditions such as hyperactivity yet also fatigue is because copper is needed to make Adenosine Triphosphate (ATP) which is pretty much chemical energy in the body. When you sprint after a thief, it is ATP that is used up, all ten seconds worth of it anyway to supply fast energy to the body. When there is excess copper in the body, a chemical chain reaction occurs which causes deficiency like symptoms simultaneously to excess symptoms. This means that copper cannot get into the cells to make ATP, which in turn causes a build-up of toxic copper in the blood stream.

Copper in this form in the blood will cause all the symptoms listed above. To find out if you have a copper imbalance you'll need to take a hair analysis test which you can purchase online. Why hair analysis? Because hair an extremely metabolically active tissue! It can most easily give you an accurate reading as to your overall health, especially when it comes to vitamin and mineral deficiency or excess.

We'll talk about how copper builds up in the body later on (Causes and Cures of Fatigue), where exactly it comes from and most importantly how to prevent copper build ups.

Seasonal Affective Disorder (SAD)

SAD, also known as seasonal depression is something which affects many people all over the world. Around 20% of Irish people are said to suffer from SAD and around 10% of Americans, although data on exact numbers have disagreed. It is known to effect women more than men, sorry ladies.

So what is SAD? As the name suggests, sufferers of SAD become depressed and fatigued in those cold winter months when there is not as much light as during the summer months.

The discoverer of SAD, Norman E Rosenthal M.D. wrote a wonderful book on the condition [21] and suggested treatments for it too. He realised that he became depressed living in New York throughout the winter months, something which he'd never experienced while living in South Africa. It was also found that the higher up the northern hemisphere, the more prevalent the condition. Of course, there is a reduction in daylight hours the more northern you get.

SAD therefore is another condition you should rule out by taking a trip to the doctors. Diagnosis normally involves a few questions, trying to figure out when and how bad the patient's depression and fatigue is during the winter months as compared to the rest of the year.

Treatment is fairly easy and straightforward. The most common being increased exposure to daylight, spending more time outside and even using mirrors to reflect more sunlight at the patient while he/she sits working at their desk. Light therapy is perhaps the most well known treatment for this condition and many thousands of light therapy units are sold every year. Light therapy simply uses a bright light placed near the sufferer to make them more alert and awake. It works and people swear by it!

Section 2

Symptoms of Fatigue

In this section we're going to talk about some of the effects and symptoms of fatigue, many or even most you'll be familiar with. Being tired for vast periods of the day is not the only effect of fatigue, it does indeed have a wider impact on our lives.

I'll also point out here that we will not always suffer from our symptoms all the time; they will of course come and go. Some days we will suffer from any number of symptoms whereas on other days we will feel fantastic.

Fatigue

When you picked up this book, it was because you wanted to cure your fatigue. But I'm sure in many cases that fatigue will not be the only symptom you'll be experiencing.

Fatigue however is the big one and most likely the symptom that is having the largest effect on your life.

Fatigue, lethargy and exhaustion are all essentially the same thing. This is the feeling of being tired at many points throughout the day, often for prolonged periods. It makes us feel weak; both physically and mentally. Often we cannot muster the energy to walk up the stairs, carry out any chores or even have a conversation with somebody. The thought of going out for a night out at a few bars sounds draining and so we pass up on our social invitations.

Fatigue is what we get when we exercise and that is normal and in fact is the whole point of exercising. However the feeling of fatigue when we're at our desks trying to work is something that shouldn't be there at all and it blights many lives.

There are two types of fatigue; physical fatigue and psychological fatigue.

Physical Fatigue

This is where you are unable to carry out a physical activity such as lifting a weight or climbing a set of stairs; whereas in normal everyday situations you'd have no problems with the task. This is common while working out as we already know. If for example, you're at home and you are too fatigued to vacuum the floor, then you would be physically fatigued.

Psychological Fatigue

This is where the mind goes into semi-sleep mode. However, this is not to say you are actually tired because this doesn't necessarily have to be the case. In most instances somebody who is psychologically or mentally fatigued would have impaired concentration levels and would not be able to think clearly. This could be very dangerous if you were driving. But it can also be incredibly difficult getting any studying done or staying single minded on a task you're carrying out.

Being fatigued can trap us in a vicious circle. If we are too tired to exercise then we become overweight. This in turn will cause us to become even more fatigued when we try to exercise.

Hopefully, fatigue will be your only symptom, in which case in the vast majority of cases the strategies you'll find in this book will change your life.

Stress

We need stress in small doses, it does after all get us out of bed. In small doses, stress can actually give us energy. However too much stress is one of the symptoms of fatigue.

Stress is a huge subject and can be a book all on its own. In fact many books have been written on combatting stress which many people have labelled 'The silent killer!'

Stress can be defined as being "subject to pressure or strain!" Unfortunately in today's modern world there are more things to stress us out than ever before. We have huge work problems, especially in today's climate, traffic that never seems to move, which in turn stops us from hitting our work targets. We have stress at home with the family and we have financial stress as well.

You can only pull a rubber band so far and eventually it will snap! Stress is the tension that keeps on pulling on that rubber band.

There are many symptoms to being stressed. The interesting thing to note is that fatigue is one of those symptoms. Once again, if you feel fatigued you will become stressed, which in turn will cause more fatigue. Also if you suffer from stress, you will feel fatigued which will cause even more stress.

Clearly it's beginning to look like everything is related to each other and we need to take an overall approach to our health, or how should I say, a complete overhaul of our lifestyles to defeat these symptoms. Anyway, I'm getting ahead of myself, more on combatting strategies later on.

Take a look at these symptoms of stress and see how many you suffer from; weakened immune system which makes us vulnerable to rheumatoid arthritis, cancer and other infections, depression and anxiety, panic attacks, drug and alcohol addiction, fatigue, exhaustion and the feeling of being run down, increased irritability and negativity, problems sleeping, headaches, racing heart, weight loss or gain, muscle tension, shortness of breath, loss of libido, shakiness, difficulties concentrating, moodiness, decreased productivity, loss of sense of humour, skin disorders such as acne and hair loss.

As you can see, there are many overlapping symptoms just as there are overlapping causes. We will go into detail about how to cut stress out of your life later as it will be very important in regaining the energy and vitality that you want.

Trouble Sleeping

You'd assume that since you're suffering from fatigue you'd have no problems getting to sleep, but this serves to demonstrate the whole complexity of the condition, that there's more to it than meets the eye.

There were many times I'd leave university half way through the day and collapse on my bed, trying to get to sleep but just couldn't. I'm sure many reading this book have experienced something similar.

The thing with trying to get to sleep at random and sporadic moments during the day is that you interrupt your body's natural cycle and destroy its habit and routine. This can cause many problems when you try getting to sleep at night time.

Another problem is that when we finally do get to sleep we often end up waking up and then find getting back to sleep again difficult. This clearly creates a chain reaction of damaged sleeping patterns which is hugely responsible for us feeling so fatigued during the day.

Sleep trouble is also a big symptom of stress as mentioned earlier. When we are under stress the body produces elevated levels of cortisol. Cortisol is responsible for increasing blood sugar, supressing the immune system and aiding in fat, protein and carbohydrate metabolism. Therefore having elevated levels of cortisol will put our body in a continuous state of hyper arousal. This causes our problems and worries to race through our minds when we're trying to get to sleep and is a huge factor in keeping us awake.

Muscle/Joint Pain

This can be extremely painful and debilitating and I've spoken to many fatigue sufferers who have had muscle and joint pain. Although this doesn't occur all the time, it can be quite common and age has no bearing on it.

If you've gone to the doctor and reported this symptom then you'll be aware about how little they know and how little they can even do for you.

You do need to be honest with yourself if you have muscle and joint pain with your fatigue. Are these symptoms as frequent as your fatigue? Did they onset at the same time? If not it's possible your muscle pain could be as a result of overuse, which is the most common cause.

Headaches

We all suffer from headaches at some point, we all know the feeling. With fatigue it is possible your headaches could be caused as a result of your muscle and joint pain, causing increased stress and tightness on the muscles in your neck. This is known as a tension headache and is the main reason people get headaches. However, if stress is also a symptom you're suffering from then your headaches could also be triggered by the stress.

Poor Concentration and Memory Loss

This would be as a result of the psychological fatigue I described earlier and after fatigue this is probably the main symptom.

This brain fog can be quite dangerous if for example you are driving. But it can have a profound effect on our daily productivity levels, not being able to stay focused or concentrate on any particular task. Studying for university or carrying out complicated work tasks can become near impossible as our minds literally wonder away onto other things. We are in effect day dreaming.

When it comes to memory loss, studies have found that when we suffer from fatigue, our brains produce less dopamine, the chemical that sends signals from one side of the brain to the other. This would perhaps explain why we know what we want to say, but often struggle to get the words out when fatigued.

Painful Lymph Nodes

Humans have around 500 lymph nodes in total. They are located all over particularly under our armpits, around our groins, necks and chest. They operate as part of our immune system.

One of the symptoms of fatigue is an enlargement of our lymph nodes which causes them to become tender and painful. This is one of the reasons we get sore throats as we have lymph nodes in our throats too. That painful feeling from swallowing is in fact tender lymph nodes.

This explains how having a sore throat can often be a symptom of fatigue.

Irritable Bowel Syndrome (IBS)

Your chances of having IBS increase with age and if you've just had an infection. Females are also around 4 or 5 times more likely to suffer from IBS than men.

IBS encompasses several symptoms; stomach pain, bloating, constipation, diarrhoea and nausea. Weight loss is also common in people with IBS due in part to it being rather painful to eat coupled with a feeling of being full.

IBS is also a major symptom of stress. Once again we're finding that these conditions are indeed linked and that an overall approach to our health and well-being is needed.

Loss of Libido

This should be fairly easy to understand in that if we're fatigued we're not necessarily going to be in the sexual mood. This can have the knock on effect of damaging relationships with our partners.

The loss of libido caused by fatigue is common in both men and women.

Stress as well as fatigue can cause a loss of libido which can then in turn cause more stress, in effect creating a vicious circle.

Sensitivity

As a result of fatigue you may find yourself becoming sensitive to the light or to loud noises. These are some of the lesser reported symptoms of fatigue but they are still known to occur.

Unfortunately, being sensitive to the light can bring on headaches since your eyes will be in pain from it. It can also bring on flashes and some people say they see shadows in their periphery vision. Being sensitive to noise also has its consequences in that this can also bring on headaches.

Depression and Anxiety

One in every six Americans will suffer from depression at one point in their life. It is a huge problem that is getting worse and worse. Depression can last for years and can attack us at any time. If a person is already predisposed to depressive bouts then this increases the likelihood of it being a symptom from fatigue.

Depression is actually a symptom and cause of fatigue which again can cause a vicious circle in the sufferer. A study [5] at the University of Loannina in Greece using over 3000 test subjects found that people with depression are more likely to be fatigued and also that people with fatigue are more likely to be depressed.

The exact same thing goes with anxiety in that it is a cause and symptom of fatigue. In small doses, anxiety can give us the fire we need to get things done. If for example, we're anxious about the messy state of our homes, we would be more likely to clean it up. However in greater amounts, anxiety can cause extreme worry, emotional stress and even fear.

Section 3

Causes and Cures of Fatigue

This next section is going to make up the bulk of this book. There are many causes of fatigue and it's important you're honest with yourself and ask if any of the causes below are true to you. Clearly it's important to know the reasons why you specifically are feeling fatigued so that you can then take the necessary action that will work for you and not everybody else.

Read through this section carefully and with an open mind as the answers to feeling great throughout your future days are below.

It is my belief that prevention is better than cure and by making natural changes to your lifestyle you can make a truly huge difference. At no point below will I recommend pumping yourself full of drugs which is what many doctors would recommend if you went to them with many of the symptoms listed above.

Think of your body as a car. If you mistreat it many things can go wrong with it. In order to take care of your vehicle properly you have to clean it regularly, keep it properly serviced, keep it tanked up with fuel and drive at sensible speeds. Perhaps this is not the best analogy to use, but I hope I'm getting my point across and as I stated earlier, an overall approach to our health must be taken to cure ourselves of fatigue.

Diet and Nutrition

There are many reasons why your diet may be giving you fatigue;

- Not eating enough
- Eating too much
- Bad eating routines
- Food allergies/intolerances
- Eating bad foods
- Not eating good foods
- Vitamin deficiencies

We'll cover each of these now.

Not Eating Enough

We get our energy from food. When we don't get enough nutrition our bodies cannot create the energy we need to operate.

The vast majority of people know that breakfast is the most important meal of the day, however according to the International Food Information Council [6] over half of us regularly skip breakfast.

Being a qualified personal trainer myself and with a degree in Sport Science I know that breakfast is essential. While you shouldn't be deliberately eating an unhealthy breakfast, you can still get away with eating more unhealthily at that time because you have the rest of the day to work it off. A report by Kelloggs [7] shows that 40% of school children don't eat breakfast and this number rises as they reach their teens. The report also states that over half of all American adults don't eat breakfast!

Skipping breakfast can seriously impair your concentration and mood, stopping you from being able to think clearly. This is psychological fatigue!

The problem is with many people that they are just unable to "stomach" food that early in the morning. If that is the case with you then you should try and make a little extra effort to have a little something, no matter how small. If you can't stomach it minutes after rising from bed, then how about having something when you arrive at work!

You really do need some food in the morning to kick start your metabolism. Remember that your body has already been all night without food as it is.

If you suspect you may not be eating enough, something that will be common if depression or stress is one of your symptoms then try keeping a food diary for the period of one week. Then use this calorie calculator [8] to see what your overall calorific intake is. Remember that males need to be aiming for 2500 calories per day and the ladies 1800. By not taking in these amounts you are in effect starving yourself.

Eating Too Much

Eating too much can cause fatigue via two main mechanisms.

Firstly, we all know that eating too much causes us to become overweight and perhaps even obese if these habits carry on for long enough. Being obese is a major factor in fatigue; we have more bulk to carry around which can become tiresome, not to mention all the other problems associated with being overweight. We will cover being overweight in a later section.

However there is another big reason why eating too much can cause us fatigue. I'm talking about eating too much in any one session or meal.

Have you ever eaten a big lunch and felt tired afterwards? I'm sure you have! In fact this is the number 1 reason we feel lethargic around mid-afternoon time, after eating our lunch.

When we eat, our blood is diverted in greater quantity to our stomachs and intestines to digest the food. The more we eat, the greater the amount of blood and for longer it is diverted. This takes blood away from our muscles and from our brains; a double whammy of physiological and psychological fatigue.

The body can easily cope with small amounts of food and digest it into the bloodstream. However when it's faced with a large meal all in one go, it struggles to cope with it all. If the body can't use the energy you've just put in then it has no option other than to store it. This is what fat is; stored energy.

A study at the University of Manchester [9] has also found that after eating, high levels of blood glucose can switch off the brain cells that keep us awake. Larger meals mean even higher levels of blood glucose and even less ability for your body to cope with it.

This is why in parts of Europe; Spain in particular and also Mexico I do believe, they have siestas every day, they literally close up all businesses and have a few hours sleep, reopening later on. Have you also noticed how your Dog always takes a nap after eating? Feeling tired after eating large meals is natural, it's your bodies way of telling you to conserve your energy because it's hard at work digesting your food.

So while there may not be anything wrong with us due to this, it does however play havoc on our productivity. So what should we do?

It's obvious, but it may take a little discipline!

Which brings us to our next section.

Bad Eating Routines

With so many of us skipping eating much at breakfast or skipping breakfast altogether and then eating until we're about to burst at lunch, we're giving our bodies a starving-gorging-starving-gorging rollercoaster of a cycle. As already stated above, this clearly will cause us problems no end.

After our huge meal at lunch we'll typically not eat anything until we arrive back home and then eat another huge meal at around 7pm. Thus the cycle continues and we're out cold for the rest of the evening.

I know full well speaking to my personal training clients that this is the pattern that the vast majority of people in the western world carry out day in day out. This isn't what nature intended for us. Back when we were cave men, we'd eat at more random and sporadic times as food wasn't readily available in huge abundance, we had to eat in small amounts as and when we found it. We were hunter-gatherers.

These days, since all the food we could ever want is right on our doorsteps or already in our fridges our eating patterns have become skewed. Not only that but society also demands we eat at set times. If we work in an office, we may get a lunch hour in which to eat and that's it.

But if we want to regain our natural vitality and defeat this dreaded fatigue then we are going to have to make changes.

I'll tell you the advice I used to give my personal training clients which helped them lose weight as well as regain an abundance of energy.

Eat less but more often!

As I was saying earlier, this takes discipline! When we eat, it's sometimes hard for us to stop! Just try telling your Dog to stop eating his meal when he's only half full and then watch him have a nap straight after he disobeys you!

I'm afraid it is of crucial importance you try and discipline yourself to eat between 6 – 8 small meals a day instead of the 3 large meals.

When you cut your meals into smaller portions like that, your body can easily deal with all the energy you're putting into it and your body will store less fat as an added bonus; preventing you from becoming overweight.

Being able to do this will depend on what your individual schedule is and whether you have a job that would enable you to carry out these kinds of eating patterns. It's of vital importance you at least make an effort with this.

Food Allergies / Intolerances

Hopefully you will already know if you have any food allergies. However, if you have IBS or stomach cramps as a symptom then chances are you have an undiagnosed food allergy. You should talk to your doctor and consider having a skin or blood test to discover if you do have an allergy or intolerance to certain foods.

Common food allergies include; nuts, fish and eggs but the truth is that you could be allergic to anything. It is important that you discover your allergy, if you have one and cut it from your diet altogether.

When you eat a food to which you are allergic, you are in effect putting something foreign into your body, something your body just cannot cope with. As a result your immune system will attack your food which will make you feel sick. This takes up a lot of energy which is why you feel fatigued if you have an allergic reaction to food.

In today's world there are more and more people who are developing intolerances to certain foods. Intolerances differ from allergies because you are born with an allergy, whereas an intolerance is something you develop over time.

Common intolerances are to wheat and to dairy products. If you have a wheat or dairy intolerance and you don't know about it then common symptoms will be fatigue, watering eyes, itchiness, stomach cramps and constipation.

Why are we developing more and more intolerances? Because food manufacturers are increasingly refining raw food products; sugar, wheat etc. taking out many natural elements that our ancestors have been eating for thousands of years. Fibre typically is becoming less and less in our daily diets, something that fills us up, lowers cholesterol and keeps us healthy.

Typically 1.5% of the population suffers from wheat intolerance. If you think this could be you then a simple test with your doctor involves pricking your skin and placing wheat on the area. Then you'll need to wait and see if your skin flares up within 15 minutes. If it does then you're one of the unlucky 1.5% who'll need to cut wheat out of their diet.

If you're suffering from fatigue, then going for a health check with your doctor is something I strongly recommend and typically one of the first things they'll do is to check for allergies or intolerances.

Eating Bad Foods

It could be that you're eating bad energy sapping foods and it's causing you to feel fatigued. The food we take in effects practically everything so never underestimate its power over us. If we eat certain foods to give us energy then it makes total sense that other foods can deplete our energy too.

I've already mentioned that you should be eating frequent small meals. However you should try and resist the temptation for too many of these small meals, or snacks to be high in sugar. I know it's tempting and they are delicious but foods high in sugar only give us a temporary lift which always comes before a big fall. After the insulin has been despatched to deal with the sudden elevation in sugar, your energy levels will fall to a point below where they were originally. So you should cut out sugary snacks as much as possible. Hey, I'm not saying you can't enjoy life, we all love things that taste nice but be honest with yourself and ask how often and how many sugary snacks you're taking in.

In fact it is the rollercoaster our blood sugar often finds itself in that is one of the reasons we feel fatigued. The wider the fluctuations the greater our fatigue! Imagine that you are hungry, you'll have low blood sugar at that moment in time. Then you eat say a donut. You'll have a very sudden and very sharp elevation in blood sugar. Your pancreas will need to dispatch a large amount of insulin to deal with the blood sugar as quickly as possible, and once it has finished its work, you will feel fatigued because your blood glucose levels ran out too quickly.

In general this pattern will arise every time we eat foods high on the glycaemic index (GI). These mainly tend to be foods high in refined sugar content, not the natural sugars found in fruit for example.

People who go to the gym regularly will often eat foods high in GI as it aids recovery time. However it really is not suitable for those of us wanting a steady supply of energy throughout the day.

Here are some foods high in refined sugar and GI which you should try and reduce or cut out entirely:

- Sugar
- Industrial made juices
- Sodas, Coca Cola, Pepsi etc.
- White bread
- White rice
- Artificial sweeteners

If however, you're really unable to cut out some of your favourite sugary foods then it's always better to have them with or immediately after your meal and never as a snack. As it will then be mixed in with more slow release carbs and protein in your gut, you won't experience as large a fluctuation.

Not Eating Good Foods

On the flip side of the above, it will be obvious that it's the slow release, low GI foods that will have the opposite effect and will give your body a nice, sustained and slower supply of energy that it needs.

When eating more of these foods, coupled with eating them in smaller portions more regularly you really are getting the best of all worlds.

Here is a list of energy boosting foods which are also low in GI:

- Legumes / pulses
- Grains
- Nuts
- Kidney beans
- Beats
- Chick peas
- Whole wheat products
- Basmati rice
- Baked potatoes
- Rolled oats
- Muesli
- All Bran / Oat Bran
- Whole wheat bread
- Brown rice
- Spaghetti
- Yam

- Sweet Potatoes
- Noodles
- Vegetables – Peas, carrots, corn, broccoli, cauliflower, cabbage, mushrooms, tomatoes, lettuce, peppers, beans, onions (raw whenever possible)
- Skimmed milk
- Yoghurt
- Most fruits excluding watermelon

For your snacks or for one of your small meal portions, a Snickers bar is also great. Nutrigrain bars are a wonderful thing to eat for sustained energy. Fruit is always underrated especially bananas and if you can face it why not eat raw veggies as a snack.

Vitamin Deficiency

By having a healthy and balanced diet you minimize the chances of being deficient in any important vitamins or minerals. Simply by following the advice already above, you should not have any problems with vitamin deficiencies that could cause you to have fatigue symptoms.

However just in case, I will briefly go over how lacking certain vitamins in your diet could cause fatigue below:

Vitamin C

As well as fatigue, lacking in vitamin C can cause general weakness and irritability. You can ensure you get adequate intake by including all your usual fruit and vegetables in your diet.

Vitamin B12

Lacking in vitamin B12 can cause anaemia, which we know fatigue is a side effect of. Other symptoms of a B12 deficiency are weakness and dizziness. You can ensure you have adequate B12 in your diet from eating animal produce.

Vitamin B6

A vitamin B6 deficiency can also cause anaemia as well as skin complaints and depression. You can find vitamin B6 in meat, fish, fruit and veg.

Folate

A lack of folate in the diet can also cause anaemia and depression. The best source of folate is green vegetables, particularly green leafy vegetables.

Thiamine

Not having enough thiamine in the diet can cause fatigue, weight loss, irritability, sleep disturbances and a poor memory. Unfortunately thiamine is increasingly being taken out of our diets due to refined produce such as sugar and flour. You can take thiamine supplements or else you can find it in whole grain cereals, legumes and nuts.

The best way of ensuring your diet contains everything you need is by keeping a food diary for at least the period of a week. Then input your diary into one of the many online templates and calculators to check your vitamin, mineral and calorie intakes. If you'd like to take things one step further then you could even visit a qualified nutritionist, who will pretty much tell you to do the same things and will input your diary into their program to check you are taking in everything you should be.

Summary

- Always eat breakfast.
- Eat smaller portions.
- But eat more often.
- Try and maintain regular eating cycles and be disciplined.
- Get a food allergy / intolerance check at your doctors.
- Reduce foods high in sugar and high on the GI scale.
- Increase foods low in sugar and low on the GI scale.
- Keep a food diary to make sure you're taking in roughly 2500 calories a day if you're male or 1800 if you're female.
- Use your food diary to ensure your diet is healthy by inputting your diary into an online nutrition calculator or why not visit a qualified nutritionist.

Dehydration

Water is the source of all life! It is absolutely essential for everything. We use it every day to clean ourselves. Well we use it to clean our outsides, but do we ever consider drinking it to clean our insides?

You see, every time we eat we are dehydrating ourselves. We need to take in water to rehydrate ourselves. Only we seldom drink water with our meals. We tend to drink soda, tea or coffee. This further dehydrates us.

Anything with sugar, or more precisely glucose serves to dehydrate us and the body needs that adequate amount of rehydration in the form of water to keep everything ticking over smoothly.

It's true that the body can pull some water out from the food we eat and even from those sugary drinks too. But it is never enough to fully hydrate us and it's a known fact that the majority of us are walking around in our daily lives dehydrated the majority of the time.

This is a problem because other than causing fatigue, being dehydrated can cause us many other problems such as:

- Irritability
- Dry skin and rashes
- Low blood pressure
- Rapid heartbeat

- Fever
- Greater susceptibility to illnesses
- Brain fog, not being able to think or concentrate
- Headaches
- Pain in joints
- Poor digestion

There is also evidence [10] that dehydration is a factor in developing Alzheimer's disease.

How many of these symptoms are common to people suffering from CFS and fatigue in general? A lot is the answer!

It is clear in my mind that dehydration is one of the fundamental reasons why we suffer from fatigue!

So how can you tell if you're dehydrated?

Well the easiest way is to check the colour of your urine. If it's dark or brown then you are dehydrated! It's as simple as that! The more clear it becomes the less dehydrated you are.

But rather than simply checking out your urine you should also be honest with yourself and ask how much water you actually drink?

Now let's get one thing straight...the water in tea, coffee and fizzy drinks does not count towards hydration. In fact they count against you!

How much *water* do you actually drink? Ask yourself!

It's important we increase the amount of water we do take in, because we don't simply lose hydration from eating and drinking sugary drinks, we also lose hydration from breathing, moving, sweating and sleeping. We lose water all the time! In fact the average adult will lose around 10 cups of water a day just through every day living.

Are you replacing these 10 cups?

Being hydrated has so many other major benefits to it other than reducing the negative effects listed above, not to mention fatigue. Water cleanses your entire body. It makes your skin feel and look amazing, it in effect keeps you young.

So what is the best thing to do about it? Well that is simple! But there are right and wrong ways about keeping your body properly hydrated.

Remember that everybody is different so the amount of water we'll need will differ. But keep in mind it depends also on heat, exercise, health and age. It will also depend on your size too.

My number one rule is that I'm never thirsty! Because if you are thirsty you're already dehydrated!

I always like to keep a bottle of water next to me and I take sips from it every five to ten minutes. Just a little sip that's all it needs, but it's regular. Yes I have to go for frequent bathroom breaks but I'm no longer fatigued!

But doesn't buying bottled water cost a lot of money? Yes it does! Which is why I don't use bottled water! Well actually I use a different plastic bottle every few days and I reuse it over and over again. I use tap water to fill my water filter, I keep the filter refrigerated and I use water from that. It works perfectly! You'll read more on why I use filtered water later on (Copper Imbalance).

I must admit, I'm also a coffee and a tea drinker. So I'm not saying you need to give up these things if you enjoy them. But you will need to make the judgement call on how badly you want to beat your fatigue. The way I get round this is by making sure I drink an extra quantity and a half of water over any tea or coffee drink I have to balance it back out again.

When I go for a workout, my habit doesn't change and I don't tend to find myself gasping for a drink no matter what I do. I simply take my regular sip every few minutes. In an average day I'll probably go through ten 50cl bottles of water.

Staying hydrated is so important to beating your fatigue, it's in fact normally the first bit of advice I give to people. In fact if there is only one thing you do seriously from this entire book, it should be to drink more water.

Summary

- Ask yourself how much water you actually drink.
- Cut out or at least reduce coffee and sugary drinks.
- Take regular sips of water! One sip every ten minutes!
- Use filtered water.

Being Overweight / Underweight

We all know just how important our weight is for our overall health. It is crucial we maintain a sensible weight for our height to remain healthy. Being either overweight or underweight can have massive effects on our energy levels and therefore make us feel fatigued.

In fact, a massive study [12] of nearly 9000 subjects in 2002 found that risks of fatigue are increased significantly for underweight women or for overweight men.

We shall now look at both in a little more detail.

Being Overweight

The easiest way to see if you are overweight is by doing a body mass index (BMI) check. Simply divide your body weight in Kg by your height in M^2. If you're in America then you can still use imperial measurements; take your weight in lbs and then multiply that number by 703 then divide that number by your height in Inches^2.

You are overweight if your BMI equals 25 or above. If it's above 30 then you are classed as obese.

As we should have had drilled into our heads by now, being overweight has many negative health implications to it, which I won't get into since you're more interested in fatigue.

There are various mechanisms why being overweight or obese can make you fatigued. The most obvious being that you have more bulk to carry around which saps more of your energy when you do anything. However I've never really believed in this school of thought because as you'll discover in a later section of this book, exercise or physical activity actually gives you energy and not fatigue.

The main reason we feel fatigued when we're overweight is because our bodies have developed a resistance to insulin. In a healthy person, insulin transports glucose into the cells for use, however in many overweight people the cells become resistant to the insulin which impairs the cells ability to properly make use of it, impairing the whole process. This causes glucose and insulin levels in your bloodstream to become unbalanced which can cause diabetes. It is a known fact that 7 million Americans have undiagnosed diabetes [11].

Being overweight can cause diabetes which will cause fatigue! If this is the case with you then the cause of your fatigue possibly may not be CFS or ME but possibly diabetes. Hopefully you will not be one of the 7 million undiagnosed Americans but if you're not sure then you should have a diabetes check at your doctors.

Thankfully you can reverse the trend of insulin resistance that your body has been experiencing. All it takes is a little exercise and reverses can happen surprisingly quickly. We'll get more into exercise later on. You need to also adapt a healthier lifestyle which following the tips already given in this book will set you well on the way.

Being Underweight

People can be underweight for a variety of reasons; illness, not eating enough, bad eating habits, major change in routine, high metabolism or stress.

If your BMI is 18.5 or below then you are classed as underweight and being underweight can make you experience fatigue symptoms.

The reasons why are pretty straightforward. Underweight people suffer from fatigue because their bodies are not getting the nutrients they need to fully function.

If this is the case then you will likely be experiencing other effects of being underweight, many of which have already been mentioned; lowered immune system, hair loss, osteoporosis, possible heart failure and anaemia.

If you are underweight then you need to focus on maintaining a healthy weight particularly by eating less but more often as stated above.

Summary

- Carry out a BMI check to determine if you're under or overweight.
- If you're overweight then begin an exercise regime.
- Eat more healthy foods as stated in the Diet & Nutrition section.
- Cut out bad foods as stated in the Diet & Nutrition section.
- If you're underweight then focus on eating smaller meals more frequently to build up to a healthy weight.

Stress

Do you suffer from stress? A study in 2011 [13] using 1200 subjects found that 22% of the American population suffers from extreme stress. Also 80% suffer from some kind of stress due solely to their financial situation.

The American Institute of Stress has found that stress related illnesses costs businesses $300 billion annually due to lost productivity and sick days. That's $7500 per employee per year! It is estimated that between 75 – 90% of all visits to the doctor are stress related.

Do not underestimate the power of stress, it has not been labelled the "silent killer" for nothing! Stress can creep up on you when you least suspect it either gradually or all of a sudden.

If you suffer from fatigue, which I assume you do if you're reading this book then chances are you're like the rest of us and you suffer from some kind of stress. Remember that stress is both a symptom and cause of fatigue which makes it even more likely that stress will be an issue for you in some form.

So what exactly is stress? Perhaps the best definition is "to subject to pressure or strain." Stress occurs when we are forced to adapt either mentally, physically or both to something in the environment. When faced with this need to change, its impact can best be measured in the intensity of the feelings and emotions we experience.

As we know though, not all types of stress are bad for us. If we had literally zero stress in our lives we probably wouldn't bother getting up in the morning. Stress can be a huge motivator as long as it's in the correct doses.

However, stress in abundance is not a good thing and can cause many of the symptoms I listed in a previous section including fatigue.

So the first thing you need to ask yourself is: Do you suffer from stress? If so then you're going to need to reduce your stress levels or eliminate them entirely. But in order to do that, you are first going to need to identify your stressors. Why not write down all the things you think are causing you stress in your life. Once you've pinned down what is causing you stress, you can then target the cause head on.

There are many things in life that can cause us stress and we'll take a look at some of them now.

- Finances
- Work
- Relationships
- Traffic
- Overload

Finances

Many of us are living on shoestring budgets and this is the number one cause of stress in the world. It can be hard when we get our monthly pay cheque and it barely even covers the overdraft we're already in. This means we don't have the money to pay for any unexpected occurrence that you never know could pop up at any time. Going on a holiday/vacation is out of the question and every month the interest alone on our credit payments gets higher and higher.

Debt seems to be the way of the world. We are born owing money, we go to college or university and we have student loan debts and that's before we've even entered the workforce.

If your finances are a cause of your stress then add it to your list. You'll need to work out a plan on improving your finances. When it comes down to it there are two ways of doing it; earn more and spend less.

Are you able to put in more shifts at work, or ask for a pay rise? Are you able to put some of your old junk on ebay? What are you talents? Are you able to make money out of this in your spare time perhaps by offering private tuition? That is a great way of making extra money!

Take a look at all your monthly outgoings. Can you reduce or remove any of them? If you have gym membership, do you actually use it enough to justify it, when you could do your running outside and not on a treadmill! Do you really need that cable subscription? Can you walk instead of driving all the time?

Here's a neat trick…If you owe money to anybody, creditors for example, have you tried ringing them and asking to do a deal? Ask them if they are willing to write off the debt if you pay half right now. This works so well because many creditors never expect to get the money anyway.

I've gone a little bit beyond the scope of this book right there so I apologize but it's because it really is a big problem for many people and a contributing factor towards fatigue.

Work

The levels of stress we encounter during our working lives will differ depending on what we do. Surveys have shown that care givers and IT workers are the most stressful occupations of them all. Teachers also tend to suffer from lots of stress along with police officers.

If you work for yourself and employ other people then the pressure could be quite overwhelming. Likewise, if you're an employee and you have strict deadlines as well as a demanding boss then these could all add up to giving your stress.

Stress in the workplace is second only to financial stress in our lives. This is not surprising in today's climate where we feel we are competing with our colleagues more than ever before. We often work overtime for free in order to try and safeguard our futures and taking our work home with us is not uncommon also.

For some people, working in a job they hate could be the cause of much stress and unhappiness. Perhaps the job is not challenging enough or you work with completely negative people who always bring you down. Are you always on the phone to angry clients or are people in your office or other departments repeatedly on your case?

Have colleagues recently been laid off and you're having to take up some of their responsibilities or are you afraid for the future of your own job?

If any of these things are a source of stress for you then write them down on your list and work to try and reduce them by whatever means necessary.

Relationships

Our relationships with our close ones; friends, children, parents and of course our significant other can be a huge source of joy. However, we all know they can be a source of stress too. This is of course a good thing really because if these people didn't stress us out then it would show we didn't really care that much for them. Of course we do care, which is why they often cause us just a little bit too much stress and unfortunately this is a source of our fatigue.

Our partner can be a source of a great deal of stress and argument which means we have no place to go to get away from it for any length of time.

If our or our partner's job is a cause of stress for them then they can often bring it back home and cause even more stress for us.

When we live with a partner, it is not just our problems that can be stressors for us, but we often take on our partner's problems too.

If your relationships are causing you stress then don't simply write down "relationships" but instead try and be more specific. What are the actual little things that are causing you stress. Get to the root of the problem so you're more able to combat the source of this stress for you.

If you're wanting to get over your fatigue then you're going to need to learn to distance yourself from the extra stress that is being caused by your relationships. This doesn't mean distancing yourself from your partner but at the very least you should learn to take more walks on your own when things get a little heated. Try and work out the small problems more calmly and rationally together.

Remember that it is in your partner's best interest that you regain your vitality.

Traffic

We all know about how insane static traffic can make us. Or even worse; stop and go, stop and go traffic. It's infuriating!

Traffic is the source of a huge amount of stress in our lives, sitting in a car that doesn't move and wasting huge swathes of our lives doing nothing.

If you have to commute to work then you'll know how this feels, particularly if you work in a big city. Thousands and millions of people all converging on one place at the same time is bound to cause chaos not only to drivers but people who take public transport too. Public transport can be overcrowded, smelly and not to mention unreliable.

How much of an issue for stress is the twice daily commute to you?

Do you want to know what I did to beat this? I left a full two hours earlier than necessary, joined a gym near my work place and did my workout in the morning in an empty gym rather than a full gym during the evenings following yet another busy commute.

We'll get into exercise for beating fatigue later on but for now, if this is an option that's available to you, setting off earlier and doing something more useful with the extra time then you should do it. You'll cruise through the traffic at 06:30 rather than at 08:00.

Clearly if you have kids who need to go to school then you should consider your options. Could your partner take them to school? How about a family friend who's kids go to the same school?

Traffic is a big source of misery for many so if it is a source of stress for you then you should work out a way to beat it like I did.

You should also consider listening to some relaxing music during your commute and not the radio or what's on your iPod. Why not give Bach a chance?

Overload

Are you unable to say no to all those people asking you favours? Do you have so much on your plate right now? Work, study, church groups, relationships, errands, volunteer work etc.

All this can quite easily get on top of us so much that we end up coming to a complete stand still and doing nothing. Trust me this is quite common, it's called a nervous breakdown!

If you find there are unreasonable demands on your time and you have no time for relaxation, which everybody needs then add to your list the things that you're doing that are not absolutely essential to your present well-being.

Do you really need to help your cousin with his project at the moment or are there other things in your diary you feel you can't commit 100% to?

There's no shame in admitting you can't handle everything right now and you really don't want to burn yourself out.

We regain our energy when we relax. How much relaxation time do you get?

Work out what you can possibly cut out from your life and do it!

Other Causes of Stress

Other potential causes of stress could be a recent major change in your life such as moving house, changing careers or perhaps a new baby has just arrived.

Do you watch the news, read the papers and are constantly aware of all the troubles, dangers and crime around the world and even in your own home town?

Have you recently suffered an accident that has had a major impact or change on your life or daily routine?

Have you suffered a death of a loved one recently and you're struggling to adjust to life without them?

Really, you need to have a good think about all the things we've just spoken about. If anything, no matter how small is causing you worries or trouble, or stress for that matter then write them down on your list.

Now you need to work on ridding yourself of these stressors, or at the very least reducing them.

What can you cut out completely and what can your partner share the burden of?

Giving you treatments for stress will not work if the reasons you're stressed are still present in your life. Removing the things that stress you out is the first step in defeating stress, which clearly since I've written a large section on, I firmly believe is a root cause and symptom of fatigue.

Once you've thought about how to remove your stressors, you can and should also use some of the "cures" many of which are also cures for fatigue. By reading the tips that follow on curing you of your fatigue, you'll also be cured of your stress since so many of the techniques have dual benefits.

Summary

- Identify what is causing you stress in the following areas; finances, work, relationships, traffic and overload.
- Have a think about any other areas of your life that are causing your stress.
- Write a list of everything you think is causing you stress.
- Tackle your stressors head on by reducing or eliminating them entirely.

Copper Imbalances

Copper is essential in the production of energy, being used in the final stages of the Krebs cycle where glucose is metabolised. Copper also has many other functions in the body such as in red blood cell production and in healing the body after infections or injuries.

However, if you have an imbalance of copper, too much of it for example then this can set off a chain reaction of negative effects which can cause symptoms such as the following; premenstrual syndrome, learning disorders, skin rashes, depression, insomnia, headaches, stress and of course fatigue.

Why does all this occur? Well it is of course very complicated science stuff but here goes.

Copper in the blood needs to be bounded to certain proteins for it to do its job. When there is an excess of copper, there are not enough proteins to bind to the copper which causes an abundance in the bloodstream to build up. Unbounded copper in our bloodstreams is toxic, it also has very strong electrical conductivity. Because of this, many free radicals, the destructive molecules which damage our cells and prematurely age us are created.

With the diet of today, copper imbalances are becoming more and more common. This eventually will cause the symptoms listed above.

That is an extremely simplified version of events, but I did make a promise that I was going to keep this book nice and simple.

One well known copper researcher has labelled copper the "emotional mineral!" This is because of the large effect of emotional conditions that a copper surplus in the bloodstream can cause. These include; depression, violence, anxiety, OCD, phobias, bipolar disorders, epilepsy, Tourette's syndrome and schizophrenia.

These symptoms often return to normal, even in suicidal patients when copper levels are brought back to normal levels.

It has also been found that violence around the world correlates with copper in the bloodstream. In regions where not much red meat is eaten (red meat contains zinc, a balancer for copper) there are higher incidences of violence.

Women tend to suffer more often from a copper imbalance than men due to birth control pills which contain copper. Those who follow vegetarian diets also tend to suffer from a surplus of copper, although this is not due to the high amount of copper in vegetables, but more to the low amount of zinc in their diets from not eating meat.

However, the most common symptom of copper surplus is indeed fatigue!

Sources of Copper

So in what food today can you find copper? Well here is a short list; red meat, chicken, eggs, nuts, coconut, grains and seeds. Although yes red meat does contain copper, it is also one of the best sources of zinc, which your doctor would put you on if you had high copper content in your blood. Chicken and eggs, as well as containing copper, also contain more than enough zinc to counteract the copper.

Chocolate is one of the highest sources of copper. It is thought that copper is associated with addiction, which could explain why we get addicted to chocolate as well as other things.

You can also find traces of copper in your water due to the copper piping.

Children can be born with a copper imbalance if it is passed down from the mother.

Stress is also a big factor in a copper surplus for the reason that it seems to naturally lower zinc levels in the blood.

Foods that once contained zinc but were stripped of it, refined foods for example white rice, sugar and white flour will also be a factor in an accumulation of copper in the bloodstream.

You will also deplete your zinc levels by drinking caffeinated drinks such as coffee and soda. If you enjoy your coffee then I'm not saying you should cut it out entirely but you should certainly try and lower the amount you're taking in.

Diagnosing Copper Toxicity

If you're worried about the amount of copper in your diet, then the best thing for you to do would be to ask for a hair analysis test at your doctors. These tests are great and will give you a wonderful overview of your general health and diet. They are also non-invasive and quick to carry out.

Treating Copper Toxicity

Once you've discovered if you have a high level of copper in your blood and/or low levels of zinc to counteract the bad effects of having high copper, then it's time to work on reducing the amount of copper in your diet in combination with increasing the amount of zinc.

When it's all said and done, a normal every day diet should in the vast majority of cases bring everything back into acceptable levels. But just to make sure -

Eat more:

- Red meat
- Whole grain rice
- Whole grain corn
- Chicken
- Eggs
- Cooked vegetables

Eat less:

- Coffee
- Sugar
- Soda / Fizzy drinks
- Coconut
- Nuts
- Aspartame
- Seeds
- Chocolate

We've already spoken about the importance of drinking lots of water, in particular filtered water. By filtering your tap water, you'll be removing any excess copper found in your water supply.

You need to also work on lowering the levels of stress in your life, something you already know how to do.

This is really all you need to know in 99% of cases with regards to the copper levels in your blood. However, there are other ways to treat copper toxicity syndrome such as holistic therapies, which are also great for combatting fatigue. Of course, we'll get into these later on.

Summary

- Take a hair analysis test to discover if you have high levels of copper and/or low levels of zinc in your blood.
- Reduce the following in your diet; chocolate, coffee, soda, nuts, coconut, aspartame, seeds.
- Increase the following in your diet; red meat, chicken, eggs, whole grain rice, whole grain corn, cooked vegetables.
- Filter your drinking water and drink plenty of it.
- Reduce the stress in your life.

Smoking

I'm sure when I mentioned we'd be taking an overall approach to our health that you assumed we'd end up talking about smoking. So if you don't smoke, feel free to save yourself a few minutes and skip this section.

There are, as I'm sure you'll already be aware of, a whole host of diseases attributable to smoking. In fact fatigue for once will be the least of your worries.

No matter what your present physical condition, quitting smoking will be the most positive thing you can do for your physical health. Quitting smoking is far more important than even losing weight for your health.

I'm not going to go into a long list of diseases and conditions you can get from smoking as I'm sure you already know these and in any case, we're here to talk about fatigue.

There are actually a few mechanisms by which smoking causes fatigue.

Cigarette smoke contains carbon monoxide, a deadly and unstable gas that can latch on to anything. Your haemoglobin molecules, the pigment that makes your blood red won't stand a chance. It is haemoglobin that binds on to oxygen and transports it around the body, to the muscles and organs so they can operate and we can survive. Not only does smoking kill many of our haemoglobin molecules, it also inhibits many others that it doesn't kill. All this prevents the body from transporting oxygen around to where it's needed. This would give us the feeling of being tired and fatigued, only we also get a fair dose of nicotine when smoking too. Nicotine is a stimulant and this temporarily tricks the body into feeling awake and not fatigued. Nicotine, as well as being the addictive force in cigarettes due in part to it being a stimulant, it also makes smokers feel more awake when they really should be fatigued albeit temporarily.

Secondly, smoking takes control and regulates blood sugar levels. If a smoker is not able to smoke, perhaps he's in a building where he's not allowed to then his blood sugar levels will drop. We all know that a sudden drop in blood sugar will give the feeling of fatigue.

I'll reiterate that because cigarettes contain nicotine, a stimulant, the smoker is tricked into thinking he is alert and not fatigued, even if he hasn't eaten anything that day.

Furthermore, if you have CFS or fibromyalgia, there are several other chemicals contained within cigarettes that are known to even further exacerbate the conditions.

My Number 1 Tip

Of course if you smoke and you really want to get over your fatigue then quitting is the best option for you.

I'll be up front and warn you right now that because nicotine is a stimulant, quitting will be hard at first. You'll also feel even more fatigued because you're not getting your regular kick, although I can promise you that this will only be temporary. While your blood sugar levels are fluctuating and readjusting to not being controlled by the dreaded sin sticks you'll have to be prepared for the inevitable fatigue that's sure to follow.

It will be worth it though, not only will you increase the amount of vitality in your life but your overall health will improve in ways you've never known. This can literally turn your life around and the money you save can be put to much better use.

Summary

- If you smoke then quit! It is the single most important thing you can do for your overall health.
- Be prepared for the short term fatigue caused by the withdrawal of the stimulant nicotine.

Depression

Much like stress above, depression is also both a cause of fatigue and a symptom of fatigue.

I'm sure if you're human you know what it's like to feel down from time to time, possibly even depressed, it happens to the vast majority of us at some point in our lives.

Depression currently effects 21 million Americans every year and has huge impacts on loss of productivity for the nation as well as great personal costs.

That feeling of waking up and not wanting to get out of bed. That feeling of hopelessness. Not being able to make decisions, even tiny decisions that have no major impact on anything such as what to have for dinner or what you're going to do in the evening. Not taking pleasure in the things you used to get great joy from. Both insomnia and oversleeping are both common in depressed people. In the most extreme cases of depression, the sufferer will have feelings of or may even attempt suicide.

Depression can also have physical as well as psychological symptoms; headaches, nausea, anxiety, loss of memory, loss of appetite and of course fatigue are all very common.

Make no mistake, depression is no joke! In fact it is a serious illness that can blight a person's life and the lives of the people around the sufferer.

While yes, you can develop depression from fatigue it is also true you can become fatigued through depression, in fact this is very common. If you suffer from fatigue, it is quite possible you are also depressed to some extent.

To illustrate my point, I make reference to a fantastic study taken in Greece [5] with 3200 subjects.

The subjects were monitored for a full year. Subjects who began the study suffering from depression were more than four times likely to suffer from fatigue. While subjects who began the study suffering from fatigue were nearly three times as likely to experience depression during the course of the study.

It seems clear that depression and fatigue feed off each other like a pair of parasites!

The head researcher Dr Pertos Skapinakis, MD says "One can possibly understand how a fatigued person can start feeling psychologically distressed because of his/her condition, but the opposite is more difficult to explain!"

Whatever the causes and mechanisms behind this, which remain unknown, it is clear that the association is there!

So what do we do about this?

Well the first thing for you to do is to ask yourself if you suffer from depression! Take another look at the symptoms above!

If you are certain you don't then you can breathe a sigh of relief, you can skip the rest of this section, as your fatigue won't be caused as a symptom of depression.

However, if you suspect you are depressed and it is a factor in your fatigue then there are several therapies you can do to "snap out of it!" As I mentioned earlier, I'm not one for trying to pump you full of drugs and the vast majority of treatments for depression are indeed drug related. This is not my approach!

Treatments for Depression

If you suffer from major depression then you're reading the wrong book and you'll require greater treatments than what's listed below.

The following are all natural, drug free methods for lifting your mood, helping to beat depression relating to fatigue or fatigue relating to depression.

Exercise

Exercising is known to lift your mood albeit temporarily. In fact exercise is probably the best method for acute stress, anxiety and depression relief.

There are reasons why we feel better mentally following a heavy session at the gym or even after a nice leisurely stroll in the park. Even light exercise produces endorphins which temporarily lift our mood.

If your fatigue is so great that you can't tolerate a heavy gym session then you should at least make an effort to do something. Start with a nice easy ten or fifteen minute walk in the park and then after a couple of weeks build this up to a thirty minute walk and then go on from there.

Exercise of course, also provides a much longer and more sustaining benefit to people's self-worth, self-esteem and confidence. When we look good, we feel good!

We'll discuss exercise more in a later section.

Stay Hydrated

We've already gone heavily into the reasons why you should be staying hydrated by drinking lots of water. This can have more positive effects on your life than you can ever imagine and it's just so simple to do.

This point really needs to be drilled home and so I mention it again here!

Healthy Eating

Read again the section on diet and nutrition! A healthy diet will do so much more for you than simply help you beat your fatigue!

Sleep

Improper sleeping patterns, sleeping at sporadic moments in the day, not sleeping at night, sleeping too much or not enough are all symptoms of fatigue and depression.

We need to have a regular pattern of good sleep to beat depression and fatigue.

We'll discuss sleep in a later section.

Cognitive Therapy

Cognitive therapy, or taking away your negative thoughts and replacing them with positive thoughts are great ways of beating depression. One thing all depressed people do is maintain a negative spiral of bad thoughts which get them down which then makes them think even more bad thoughts.

The basis of cognitive thinking is that your thoughts precede your moods. So that by replacing negative thoughts with positive thoughts, you can improve your mood from negative to positive. However you can not only improve your mood but also your behaviour and physical state too.

Cognitive therapy has been shown in studies [14] to be very effective in treating depression.

Cognitive therapy includes carrying out activities, or hobbies that give you pleasure! What activity takes your mind off the negative aspects of your life, focuses you on the positive and gives you lots of pleasant associations? When you feel depressed you should carry out this activity.

When you are feeling, thinking or talking negatively to or about yourself you need to recognize that you are doing this and stop! Do not ever talk yourself down! Saying you're too fat, lazy, incompetent, stupid or boring will of course lower your mood. Instead you should focus on what's good about yourself and your achievements to raise your mood.

If you lack confidence or self-belief, then you should read the best book I've ever read on the subject of confidence [15]!

Finally, if you really want to give cognitive therapy a good go then you should seek out a professional. Ask for a referral from your doctor.

Summary

If you suffer from depressive symptoms:

- Seek a referral from your doctor.
- Exercise can provide temporary lifts to your mood.
- Exercise can also provide longer term boosts to your self-esteem.
- Stay hydrated.
- Maintain a healthy diet.
- Keep a normal sleeping pattern.
- Use cognitive behavioural therapy treatments from a qualified practitioner.

Sleep Problems

Approximately 100 million Americans suffer from some form of sleeping disorder. Fortunately the vast majority of these are extremely minor, suffering from the occasional bad night of sleep. However, of course many of these will be more serious, with every combination in between and many of these will be the cause of fatigue for many people. In fact in the Sleep in America poll of 2007 [16], 60% of women said they only get a few good nights of sleep per week.

We spend a huge amount of our lives sleeping, and if you're reading this book, then I'm sure you feel like the need for a lot more. The truth is that is not necessarily the case.

There are four fundamental bad sleeping practices that can cause fatigue:

- Not enough sleep
- Too much sleep
- Sleep disturbances
- Irregular sleeping patterns

We shall go into each of them now.

Not Enough Sleep

Not getting enough sleep, otherwise known as insomnia is the most common sleeping complaint among Americans and is a big factor in the daily fatigue we feel. It is a safe bet that if you don't get much sleep and you are fatigued throughout the day, then it is your lack of sleep which is a major factor in that.

If you only suffer from the occasional bad night sleep then this really won't be much of a problem. The problem occurs when it is more long term.

So why do we get long term insomnia?

The main reasons are as a result of some other condition we're suffering from, most notably stress! Once again, being stressed out can have a major effect on our energy levels.

I'm sure we've all had the odd sleepless night due to some big event or day that's approaching, however when we have serious problems that are causing us stress such as financial or relationship difficulties then we can quite naturally suffer from insomnia. If this is the case for you then you already know about the importance of dealing with stress from the section above.

You may also suffer from insomnia due to physical pain you're experiencing, perhaps an injury.

Another common cause of insomnia is depression, which is also another cause of fatigue (see depression).

Finally, you may also be suffering from insomnia due to some form of medication you're taking for some other condition. Birth control pills as well as some cold and flu remedies can keep you up all night long.

If you are struggling to get to sleep at night then you should first try and determine if it is due to some other condition you're suffering from, it is important to get to the root cause first. For example, if it's stress related then you need to deal with your stress rather than just popping some pills. As we've already discussed, getting rid of or even reducing your stress can have a wonderful benefit to your life.

Treatment for Insomnia

Carry out the following drug free treatments to improve your sleep:

- Drink less coffee and other caffeinated drinks.
- Quit smoking, cigarettes contain the stimulant nicotine.
- Exercise during the day or evening. If not then at least go for an evening stroll before bedtime.
- Avoid taking midday naps or snoozes.
- Go to bed at the same time every night and establish a proper sleeping routine.

- Awake at the same time every morning and establish a proper waking routine.
- Have a small snack prior to going to bed, but not too much.
- Remove noise! Close doors, turn off TV's, radios, cell phones etc.
- Experiment with white noise, a fan or soothing pan pipes on CD.
- Reduce the stress in your life.

Finally, the reasons you're not getting enough sleep may be down to sleep disturbances you're suffering from (see sleep disturbances).

Too Much Sleep

Now you're probably wondering why anybody who gets too much sleep would be suffering from fatigue! The fact is that oversleep often *does* cause fatigue! I know because I've spoken to many people who have complained that even though they are sleeping between ten and twelve hours a day, they are still tired. The person I counselled about fatigue who was getting the most sleep was wondering if his 14 hours a day was not enough! That's right! Can you believe that? A guy I know was sleeping 14 hours a day and still feeling tired!

To say that everybody sleeps every day, it really is incredible just how little is actually known about it.

However, we do know that certain things can make you oversleep. Certain medications can have that effect on you. If you feel you are oversleeping then you should check with your doctor if it is a side effect of any drugs you're taking.

Excessive alcohol and caffeine consumption can really have a big effect on oversleeping. We've all been really drunk and then found waking up the next day really hard. However, if this is a regular routine for you then you should clearly cut down on your alcohol and caffeine intake.

I've found that the majority of people who oversleep tend to be younger people, no surprise there then is there! The reason for this problem is that many people just don't have reasons for getting out of bed in the morning. School or college holidays or simply just the weekends and oversleeping can cause havoc with your body clock. If this sounds like something you can relate to then try getting a part time job for the holidays and weekends, or simply get yourself a new hobby, preferably something that involves physical activity.

That brings us to physical activity. It is also a great cure for the early morning blues. If you can't pull yourself out of bed in the mornings then you should exercise late in the evening. This really does help to give you more firepower in the morning.

Try and get into a regular sleeping pattern! Go to bed at the same time every night and set your alarm for a respectable hour. Station your alarm at the opposite side of the room and put it on full blast so you're forced to get up to turn it off. Then remain disciplined and don't go back to bed. I also find that sleeping with your curtains open to allow the day light in can help a lot.

All you really need is anywhere between seven and eight hours of sleep a night. Any more than that and you're setting your body off into irregular routines that it won't be able to get used to.

Sleep Disturbances

As we know, sleep disturbances in both men and women are really common. To have a good night sleep that will make us feel invigorated the following day, it's not just about the length of your sleep but also the quality of your sleep.

Having eight hours of constantly interrupted sleep every night would have the same negative effect as only getting three or four hours sleep.

There are many types of sleep disturbances out there such as; insomnia, hypersomnia (the opposite of insomnia), narcolepsy and probably the most common - sleep apnea which we'll touch on below.

However before we do that, I'll also point out that many sleep disturbances are man made and you should do your best to ensure that human disturbances are minimized. These would include noisy children, noisy partners, snoring partners, TV's, cell phones, traffic, neighbours, music and anything else you can think of. If there is anything that is waking you up frequently throughout the night, then get them to put a sock in it!

Sleep Apnea

18 Million Americans suffer from sleep apnea, it's actually fatal in 38,000 cases each year. If you suffer from sleep apnea you may not even be aware of it, as it's often something that's pointed out to the sufferer by a partner.

Sleep apnea is basically when you stop breathing while you sleep, causing you to wake up. Most times this will happen without you even knowing it.

It is very common in people who snore and more common in those who're overweight. Smokers are also at greater risk from sleep apnea than non-smokers.

If you suspect this is a problem for you then you should go and see your doctor. You can be diagnosed via a polysomnogram which is a sleep test.

Usual treatments include surgery to unblock airways but going on a weight loss program will also help a lot too, not to mention quitting smoking.

Irregular Sleep Patterns

Unfortunately, having irregular sleeping patterns may not be something you'll be able to do very much about.

This all depends on your job and routine. Perhaps you work shifts, occasionally at night, sometimes at day so you have to sleep whenever you can. Or maybe you have a new baby in your family and you have to give consideration to the little guy, not to mention being woken up by the baby.

Whatever the reason, by not allowing your body a regular routine of good quality sleep, you can cause yourself fatigue during your waking hours. This has been proven in a study [17] involving students in Taiwan.

The key, as I've already mentioned is to simply establish a good routine of seven or eight hours sleep a night, scheduled at the same time every day.

It is understandable that this may not be something everybody will be able to do because of their job. If this is the case with you then you should instead focus on quality sleep while you can by following the advice already given.

For those who're able to take the advice in this section you should really try and concentrate on a routine of high quality sleep, this should also apply to the weekends.

Your routine shouldn't simply be for your sleeping hours however. Try and establish a routine for the hours preceding bed time. This should include eating a small snack at the same time before bed, ideally an hour before sleeping. Why not have a hot bath after your snack and finish off by reading your favourite book for half an hour.

Within a short space of time your body should get used to this new routine and sticking to it should be easy.

Summary

If you're not getting enough sleep:

- Reduce the stress in your life.
- Consider if you're taking medication that's keeping you awake.
- Reduce your caffeine and alcohol intake, particularly late in the evening.
- Quit smoking.
- Exercise more.
- Avoid midday snoozes.
- Establish a regular sleeping routine.
- Create a comfortable sleeping environment by reducing noise.

If you're getting too much sleep:

- Consider if any medication you're taking is causing you to sleep too much.
- If you're a student, have something to wake up for! Get a new active hobby!
- Exercise in the evenings.
- Establish a regular sleeping routine and stick to it.

If you suffer from sleep disturbances:

- Create a comfortable sleeping environment, reduce noises and distractions and promote white noise.
- Turn off the cell phone!

- Visit your doctor regarding anything more serious such as sleep apnea, narcolepsy, night terrors or restless leg syndrome.

If you have irregular sleep patterns:

- Establish a regular sleeping routine and stick to it, even at weekends.
- Establish a pre bedtime routine.
- Aim for seven to eight hours per night.

Alcohol Intake

Having a high alcohol intake can cause fatigue via a number of different mechanisms which we will discuss below:

- Anaemia
- Dehydration
- Depression
- Sleep disruption
- Withdrawal symptoms

Anaemia

We spoke about anaemia briefly above as being one of the conditions you could possibly have if you suffer from constant fatigue. Anaemia, along with other conditions should be ruled out by your doctor.

Anaemia is where there is an abnormally low level of red blood cells or haemoglobin molecules to transport oxygen around the body to the muscles and organs. Factors which can cause a reduction in red blood cells or decrease their efficiency are low iron intake, a recent large loss of blood, smoking or drinking.

It's true that through regular heavy drinking, it's possible for anaemia to be triggered and as we know, anaemia can cause fatigue [18].

As we know, red blood cells are produced in the bone marrow and studies have found that the bone marrow of heavy drinkers can become impaired.

Dehydration

Alcohol is a major cause of dehydration. I'm sure you've seen the colour of your urine following a night of heavy drinking. As we know from an earlier section, being dehydrated is one of the major causes of fatigue.

It doesn't matter if you are a light drinker, drinking only on occasions or if you're an alcoholic who drinks every day. By taking in alcohol, the water in your blood that is displaced will need to be replaced to prevent dehydration from occurring.

This is a lot easier to do if you only drink on the odd occasion. Simply take in extra water to account for the increase in alcohol. You should also make sure you eat before a night out drinking, or have alcohol with your meal and you should try your best to drink water between alcoholic drinks.

By no means would I ever tell you to give up alcohol, having fun and a social life, but if you suffer from fatigue then you should take sensible drinking into account.

If you're an alcoholic then I don't think reading this book would be the immediate answer to your problems and more emphasis should be placed on giving up, or reducing your alcohol intake.

Depression

As we know, depression can cause fatigue! See the section on depression for more on this.

However there are disagreements as to whether heavy alcohol drinkers become depressed or depression causes people to become heavy drinkers. It's a bit like the what came first the chicken or the egg analogy.

Some studies have indeed shown that depressed people turn to drink in order to "self-medicate" and ease their woes, however there are other studies that have shown heavy drinking can also lead to depression [19, 20].

Whichever may be true, the link to alcohol intake and depression is there and there is no doubt at all that depression can lead to heavy fatigue.

Sleep Disruption

As we know, irregular sleeping patterns, having disrupted sleeping schedules, under as well as over sleeping can cause us to become fatigued.

Alcohol affects our sleep!

Have you ever tried getting up in the morning while hung over? This can then have knock on effects over the next few days trying to get your body clock back on track and in the meantime you'll be fatigued and have practically zero energy to do anything. While hung over, we tend to rise from bed late in the evening, or simply sleep through the entire day and following night.

I know the temptation to have the occasional big night out with heavy drinking and a few friends is high and I'd never tell you to give that up. If however this is a several times a week thing for you, perhaps you're a student (I remember my student days, just) then this could be one of the primary reasons for your fatigue.

Withdrawal Symptoms

Becoming sober following a long period of alcoholism will play all kinds of havoc on your system.

Alcohol is a sedative, another reason it can cause you fatigue and of course drowsiness. However when your body is not getting this addictive sedative that it needs, withdrawal symptoms will inevitably follow. It is the same as giving up smoking or anything else addictive.

The symptoms from giving up alcohol following an addiction would be insomnia, cravings, mood instability and of course fatigue. These symptoms can last for many months however, rest assured it will become gradually easier as time passes by.

Also, the heavier the drinker, the worse the withdrawal symptoms are likely to be.

Drinking should be fun and not something you depend on. Clearly, a sensible attitude to drinking is what is necessary to ensure it does not become a reason for causing you fatigue.

Summary

- Maintain sensible drinking practices.
- Always eat before a big night of drinking.
- Try and remain as hydrated as possible by drinking water between alcoholic drinks.

Physical Activity

When reading this book, much of the advice given is simply about living a healthy lifestyle. I believe that healthy living is the key to vitality and being full of energy and so of course, exercise is a big part of all that.

But you're probably thinking that exercise will take away your energy, not give you it, but in fact the opposite is true.

To prove this, I'm going to refer to a study that was conducted at the University of Georgia in 2008 [22].

The study took place over a period of six weeks with 36 adults who'd complained of fatigue. Other than the fatigue, they were healthy. The subjects were split up into three groups; a low intensity workout group, a medium intensity workout group and a non-exercise group. The subjects who were in the exercise groups had to attend the exercise lab three times a week for the following six weeks. The subjects were measured on their vigour and fatigue states.

After six weeks it was found that subjects in both exercise groups felt reductions in their fatigue, which were also unrelated to their previous fitness levels.

In case you're curious, the group who exercised in the low intensity group experienced the greater benefits to their feelings of fatigue.

So there you have it! Take a look at the study yourself and see what you think.

But does this really come as any real shock or surprise? That exercising over a long period of time has benefits to our overall health and to our overall energy levels in particular.

The great thing about that study is that you really don't need to exercise all that vigorously to achieve the benefits. In the study, both exercise groups exercised on stationery bicycles, with the low intensity group exercising extremely leisurely, the equivalent of riding a bike on level ground, whereas the medium intensity group rode on a bit of an incline.

This goes to show that you can achieve great improvements to your energy levels over a long period of time simply by getting outside and doing something nice and light such as cycling on level ground or going for a walk in the park.

So what are the reasons behind exercise giving you energy when common sense should dictate exercise should take it away from you?

Well the truth is that exercise has so many benefits, that I'm sure you're aware of that it could be through a number of mechanisms. The most likely reason being that exercise improves your entire cardiovascular system, making it more efficient at carrying oxygen around in your blood to the working muscles and organs.

Exercise, even very light aerobic exercise will increase the number of red blood cells and haemoglobin molecules in your bloodstream. The heart increases in size and becomes more efficient, better enabling the pumping of the blood around the body. What's more, the number of mitochondria in the cells increase and they also grow larger. Mitochondria are the organelles in cells which are responsible for creating energy. They are known as our cells "power houses."

I could go on and on! But I hope you're beginning to see why even doing a small amount of light exercise every other day will have serious long term benefits to your overall energy levels.

If you're reading this book and you already have an active lifestyle then carry on doing what you're doing, I'm sure you already appreciate that exercise not only gives you energy in the long term but in the short term as well.

So why is this?

Again, there are many reasons for this!

Exercise releases endorphins, the same feel good chemical which is released when you're excited or in orgasm. They are produced by the pituitary and the hypothalamus in the brain and so are responsible for the natural high you experience often for hours after exercising.

Exercise is also a great stress killer, we've spoken at large about stress and its effects on your energy levels. In addition, exercise also fights against acute depression, another thing that can cause fatigue. We've also spoke at length about that! Finally, exercise helps you sleep better and we know how important a good night sleep is to our energy and overall health.

So there you have it, exercise will give you energy in both the short and long term. It really is a win-win situation.

So if you're presently a sedentary individual, what am I suggesting you do?

Firstly, if you're overweight, you should first visit your doctor to ensure it's safe for you to begin an exercise regime.

Once you've been given the thumbs up, you should join a gym and speak to a qualified personal trainer. They will put you on a program to suit your needs, wants and goals.

It is recommended that you carry out a minimum of three or four, thirty to forty minute light exercise sessions per week. These can involve your walk to work or getting the shopping. Incorporating exercise into your lifestyle should be one of your aims.

If you don't presently exercise, then this should be one of your priorities in order to destroy your fatigue once and for all.

Summary

- It is proven that exercise increases energy levels and decreases feelings of fatigue both short and long term.
- If you don't exercise, check with your doctor that it's safe for you to do so.
- Join a gym and hire a personal trainer.
- You should exercise a minimum of three times per week for 30 – 40 minutes.
- Incorporate exercise into your lifestyle by walking to work and to other places.

Poor Workplace Practices

Hopefully having a workplace that is contributing to your fatigue levels will only count for a minority of people reading this book, but I know that working in certain environments can play havoc with your energy levels. I've spoken to many people over the years who've had to grin and bear it in order to bring the money home.

Workplace practices that can cause fatigue include the following:

- Long shifts
- Irregular shift patterns
- Night shifts
- Heavy or manual labour
- Loud environments
- Hot environments
- Boring environments

We'll talk briefly about each one now:

Extra Long Shifts

You don't need to be a rocket scientist to understand why working long hours will cause fatigue. Long shifts give you little or no time to do anything else such as exercise and de-stress, they can also cause your body clock to get messed up.

Irregular Shift Patterns

Working nights one week and then days the next could mean your body is not able to adjust to the changes in work patterns. This can cause severe stress and fatigue as well as mess up your sleep schedule.

Night Shifts

There are reasons we're supposed to work during the day time! Our bodies naturally shut down over night, just like they have done for thousands of years. If you work during the night then your body is fighting evolution.

Heavy or Manual Labour

Carrying out repetitive tasks that use up a lot of energy will cause us to become exhausted. The best therapy for this is plenty of short breaks with intakes of food and don't forget the water.

Loud Environments

Working in a loud place such as a train station or in a factory could cause us fatigue through increased levels of stress and headaches.

Hot Environments

Working in a hot kitchen or factory can of course send you to sleep on the spot! These days, in many countries there is legislature regarding working in hot environments and your rights. You should find out what they are and ensure you're getting the proper breaks and adequate hydration throughout the day.

Boring Environments

Well this is obvious! And unfortunately there's not much anybody can do to make fun of a boring work environment to keep you awake save for an iPod and your favourite songs.

If any of the above apply to you then it's important that you isolate the actual reason why your job is causing you fatigue.

Are you able to change this in any way? Perhaps work in a different department? Change your work environment somehow or perhaps even, if worst thing comes to the worst change jobs. When it's all said and done, if your job is affecting your health then perhaps you should be in a different job.

Section 4

Extra Energy Boosting and Fatigue Killing Strategies

All the strategies above are concerned with your lifestyle! By making small adjustments that everybody should be doing you really can become that high energy person you really should be. Everything you read in the section above will not just kill your fatigue but will make you an overall healthier and happier person.

This next section is not concerned with your lifestyle, things you may be doing wrong in your life that is causing you fatigue, but is instead going to talk about what you could be doing extra to boost your energy through a range of different methods and techniques.

Everything you've read above is what I highly suggest you do! Everything you read below are optional extras to give you that much needed advantage! While not necessary, I would suggest you try a few of them out to see if they make a difference for you.

Have Goals for the Coming Day

When we set goals for ourselves and physically write our goals down on a sheet of paper, we are setting our minds in gear towards getting them accomplished no matter what.

By having this anticipation of the forthcoming activities, our minds will produce the necessary energy in order to get them done. Because we are looking forward to a list of things we know we have to do that day, our minds will ensure we are perky and in a good shape to complete them.

Have you heard of the saying "mind over matter?" This is how our minds can command our bodies, through positive thinking. This is how our state of minds can have a positive influence on the amount of energy we have.

By doing the opposite and not reinforcing the message to the brain that you have a busy day ahead, your body will not keep aside the energy it needs to get you through it.

So make sure you pack your day full of activities you want to get done and goals you want to achieve and write them down on paper the night before or while you eat your breakfast in the morning.

Try it out and observe how you feel so much more positive for the duration of the day.

Deep Breathing Exercises

We breathe on average 20,000 times in a single day, yet how much emphasis do we ever actually place on quality breathing?

When we breathe we are passing oxygen throughout our bodies, which gives us energy. We are also getting rid of carbon dioxide, a toxic gas that would suffocate us if left in our blood. Given those two simple facts, it's amazing we don't put more thought into good breathing techniques in order to alleviate fatigue, or for simply living in a healthy way in general.

I've had many personal training clients say to me that they always try and induce a yawn prior to starting a set of weights at the gym. This was something I could relate to. When we yawn, we are taking in a big burst of oxygen, a big burst of energy to get us through lifting those heavy weights.

By spending a little bit more time concentrating on our breathing, we can give ourselves a lot more energy for the day ahead.

There are reasons why many doctors now simply advise their patients to practice deep breathing exercises. There are many positive effects such as; relieving stress, lowering blood pressure, improving the quality of your sleep, improving circulation and of course it will raise your energy levels.

By controlling your breathing and slowing it down a couple of times a day for a few minutes, you can reap all those rewards.

So how do you do it?

Well feel free to take a look at some of the many great deep breathing resources available on the web. But here's one you can try now:

- Find a quiet room with no distractions.
- Sit down cross legged and open up your chest.
- Inhale slowly, taking around 6 – 8 seconds.
- Hold for 15 – 20 seconds.
- Exhale for 10 – 15 seconds.
- Repeat at least 10 times.
- Do this twice a day.

Give this a go and see how you feel!

Meditation

Meditation has been used for thousands of years for a whole range of purposes.

There are many studies that show meditation is great for relieving stress, reducing depression and anxiety, help improve sleep, increase energy and vitality as well as a lot more on top of that.

It has even been found in one study [23] that meditation helps reduce the symptoms of fibromyalgia which as we know includes fatigue as a symptom.

Please do not overlook the power of meditation simply because it seems silly. Meditation can and should be a powerful tool you use to enhance the overall quality of your life and in particular to reduce stress and fatigue.

So how does meditation do all these great things?

Well you are training your body to relax! When we relax, we lower the levels of cortisol being produced. Cortisol is known as the stress hormone because it is released when we become stressed. High levels of cortisol in the blood is associated with; fatigue, increased blood pressure, stress, miscarriage as well as weight gain.

It has to be stressed that meditation is not a cure for any of these symptoms, but it has been known to be relieving.

Added benefits of meditation are that it can really help you to focus and take your mind off your problems.

There are no real downsides to meditation other than it can take time to get good at it and daily practice can be up to 20 minutes which you may not always find easy to fit in. It doesn't however cost any money unless you decide to take a class, something which would be recommended when starting out.

Relaxation Music

We all love listening to music, but when we have fatigue, there is a difference between listening to heavy metal in the car on the way to work and listening to something a little more soothing.

Studies [24] have indeed shown that listening to music can reduce stress, anxiety and fatigue. Listening to soothing music has also been shown to help you get a good night sleep, reducing the effects of insomnia which as we know can further help fight against fatigue.

How does all this work? Well music makes us feel wonderful and positive. It also calms us down, relaxes our muscles, reduces stress, blood pressure, heart and respiratory rate. It works in a very similar way as meditation does.

However you do need to make sure the music is soothing and relaxing. Bach has been known to work very well for this purpose. I personally have always liked pan pipes.

I'm sure you'll already know what works well for you! Listen to something soothing in the mornings and before you go to bed at night.

Yoga

We've already covered the positive effects of exercise on fatigue, so it should come as no surprise that yoga would have similar positive effects. However, I would like to focus on yoga for a little bit due to its low impact and easy nature. While many people may struggle to go for a long jog, trying out yoga is fairly simple and attending a class will be extremely enjoyable.

Yoga has been shown to have positive effects on fatigue in various studies, here's one of them [25]. It has also been shown to reduce depression and stress as well as being great for focusing attention, deep breathing and relaxation. Once again, this sounds similar to mediation and we've already spoken of the great benefits of that.

In fact many doctors these days are recommending yoga to patients with CFS, ME, Fibromyalgia or simply just symptoms of fatigue. If you have never tried it then it's something I strongly recommend you have a go at.

Consider buying a few good books on the subject and learning the yoga positions. Or better yet you could join a few classes in your local area. The latter would be preferential as you will be given actual guidance.

The key is to start off slowly, using only a few yoga positions at a time and then building up from there. Before long you'll really enjoy it and you can incorporate your yoga, meditation, deep breathing exercises and relaxation music into one.

So what are the mechanisms behind yoga being so effective? Here they are:

- Yoga reduces stress by decreasing the amount of cortisol in your blood.
- It is a gentle workout with the de-stressing, depression fighting and fatigue combatting elements that go with it.
- Helps you concentrate on your breathing.
- The gentle stretching of the muscles removes toxins and improves flexibility.
- Gentle exercise is great for getting a good night sleep.

Is there a better, cheaper, more fun or more effective method of beating fatigue? I don't think so!

Massage Therapy

As well as being extremely enjoyable, massage therapy has all kinds of benefits to the human body:

- It can help sports injuries.
- Relieve acute pain.
- Decrease depression.
- Cure headaches.
- Enhance immune functionality.
- Remove toxins.

It has also been shown [26] to reduce anxiety, depression, pain as well as fatigue in as little as one session!

Read that last paragraph again!

Following the first session, in the same study, symptoms continued to alleviate for the remainder of the five week study!

I myself can testify, albeit anecdotally that my headaches from tight shoulder and back muscles were reduced in a big way after only one session of massage and then after another two, my headaches (from overarching at a computer screen) had completely vanished.

There are many types of massage; Indian head massage, Swedish massage, Thai massage, sports massage, remedial massage as well as aromatherapy massage. The best thing to do would be to speak to a qualified therapist and let her or him make their recommendation to you.

Massage is yet another thing that many doctors are recommending for the treatment of stress and fatigue, and it's something that I myself, writing this book am recommending to you too.

Conclusion

The first thing you should be doing when faced with fatigue is to rule out any medical condition you may have. I'm afraid this should involve a trip to the doctor.

If you do have one of the medical conditions listed in the first section of this book then the best thing to do is to take your doctor's advice. The advice I have given in this book, natural, healthy, everyday lifestyle advice will still do amazing things for you.

After going to the doctor and CFS, ME etc have been ruled out, it's likely you're just fatigued like the majority of the rest of the population will experience in their lives.

Following the lifestyle advice in this book is all you need to know to rebuild your vitality and banish your fatigue to your personal history book forever. It really is that simple!

I understand that you're probably not going to be able to markedly change your entire lifestyle overnight. But you can quite easily concentrate on a few of the more important things at first. Then over the following weeks, incorporate more positive lifestyle changes into your everyday life.

The very first thing you should be doing is ensuring you remain hydrated. That really is number 1 in fighting fatigue. You need to also quit smoking! Concentrate on those two things first.

Once you have done that then slowly begin an exercise regime and improve your diet exactly as I have suggested.

Then you should concentrate on dealing with any high levels of stress which you may have. Believe me, that's a big one that should not be underestimated! Then try and improve the quality of your sleep!

Simply by doing these things, not only will you have energy flooding through you like never before, but your overall health will be incredible.

From then on you should try out the other techniques I listed later on just for fun! I especially recommend massage, it works wonders.

Please let me know how you get on! I would love to know about your success stories and I may even include them in a 2nd edition to motivate other sufferers of fatigue. If you leave a review on the Amazon sales page and you have an email address listed on your Amazon reviewer profile then I will contact you.

I wish you the very best of luck and vitality!

References

1. http://www.bmj.com/content/333/7568/575
2. http://www.ncbi.nlm.nih.gov/pubmed/7916407
3. http://www.bbc.co.uk/news/health-12252813
4. http://www.amazon.com/gp/product/B00740GHB0/ref=as_li_ss_tl?ie=UTF8&tag=kindle0b38-20&linkCode=as2&camp=1789&creative=390957&creativeASIN=B00740GHB0
5. http://www.psychosomaticmedicine.org/content/66/3/330.full
6. http://www.foodinsight.org/
7. http://kelloggs.mediaroom.com/index.php?s=43&item=346
8. http://caloriecount.about.com/
9. http://www.newscientist.com/article/dn9272-why-we-need-a-siesta-after-dinner.html
10. http://lisa-c-deluca.suite101.com/causes-prevention-of-alzheimers-a72985
11. http://ndep.nih.gov/diabetes-facts/index.aspx
12. http://arno.unimaas.nl/show.cgi?fid=2118
13. http://www.apa.org/news/press/releases/stress/2011/final-2011.pdf
14. http://www.ncbi.nlm.nih.gov/pubmed/9574861
15. http://www.amazon.com/mn/search/?_encoding=UTF8&keywords=confidence%20for%20men%20charlie%20valentino&tag=kindle0b38-20&linkCode=ur2&qid=1333555019&camp=1789&creative

=390957&rh=i%3Aaps%2Ck%3Aconfidence%20for%20men
%20charlie%20valentino

16.
http://www.sleepfoundation.org/sites/default/files/Summ
ary_Of_Findings%20-%20FINAL.pdf

17. http://www.biomedcentral.com/1471-2458/9/248

18. http://pubs.niaaa.nih.gov/publications/arh21-1/42.pdf

19. http://www.ipass.net/a1idpirat/Alcoholism-
Depression.html

20.
http://www.ncbi.nlm.nih.gov/pubmed/19255375?dopt=A
bstract

21.
http://www.amazon.com/gp/product/1593851162/ref=as
_li_ss_tl?ie=UTF8&tag=kindle0b38-
20&linkCode=as2&camp=1789&creative=390957&creative
ASIN=1593851162

22.
http://content.karger.com/ProdukteDB/produkte.asp?Akti
on=ShowAbstract&ArtikelNr=116610&Ausgabe=235759&P
roduktNr=223864

23.
http://www.fammed.wisc.edu/sites/default/files/webfm-
uploads/documents/outreach/mindfulness/res-
mindfulness-fibromyalgia.pdf

24. http://www.ncbi.nlm.nih.gov/pubmed/20635523

25.
http://ukpmc.ac.uk/abstract/MED/15055096/reload=0;jse
ssionid=tHh7BlnT2TepAXX9hqAA.4

26. http://psycnet.apa.org/psycinfo/2000-14136-002

Case Study with Andrea Parker (33), Professional Dancer.

James Driver: When did you first notice you were suffering from fatigue?

Andrea Parker: Since I was 21. Which was around 12 years ago!

JD: How did this feel to you and how did it affect your everyday life?

AP: I used to have really bad lower back ache, especially when I was walking and I always just felt like I had less energy than everybody else. I could never understand why this was because I'd always had a good diet from childhood.

JD: Were you suffering from any other symptoms?

AP: I had swollen glands in my neck, they'd get really bad for no reason. Quite often I'd get really confused, I didn't have any infections that I knew of at that time although later it was revealed I had a tooth infection which I eventually had removed.

JD: And your fatigue remained even after the tooth was removed?

AP: Yes it did!

JD: How were your sleeping patterns back then? Were they affected by your fatigue and did you succumb to having afternoon naps?

AP: No it didn't get to that stage but when I woke up in the morning, I really felt terrible and my brain just couldn't function at all. I just felt so groggy, almost like having a hangover. I used to struggle to get going in the mornings and that was pretty much most mornings.

JD: How about getting to sleep at night? Was that ever a problem for you?

AP: No I've never really had sleep problems.

JD: What were your meal patterns like back then? Were they infrequent large meals or were they more regular small meals?

AP: It was usually just the three meals a day; breakfast, lunch and evening meal.

JD: Did you ever skip breakfast?

AP: I never skipped breakfast ever. I couldn't function if I didn't have breakfast.

JD: Have you always considered yourself healthy? Have you always had a healthy diet?

AP: I've always had a healthy diet and have been aware of what I eat. I've always tried to avoid food with chemicals in and I've always tried to eat as organic as possible.

JD: After how long did you finally visit the doctor?

AP: Well at first I didn't realise it was fatigue that I had, I just thought that everybody else was the same as me. So I didn't actually see a doctor until 8 years into it, that was when I started to lose my voice, I thought that was down to my dance teaching at first. But then when I started to rest my voice box I still tended to lose my voice quite frequently.

JD: So when you finally went to the doctor, did he perform any tests on you at all?

AP: He sent me to the hospital after a couple of visits when it didn't seem to go away. They put a camera down my throat and had a look at my voice box. They said there was absolutely nothing wrong with it and made out like I was making it up. They didn't see anything wrong with me at all. I just went away completely confused and gradually got my voice back again, then lost it again. I just couldn't pin point what was triggering it, it didn't seem to be food, it wasn't what I did for a living, it was just completely confusing. That was when I went to see alternative therapists.

JD: We'll get into alternative therapists soon. First, tell us what you tried that didn't work for you.

AP: Over the years I've tried glucosamine and vitamin E. Vitamin E did tend to help me a little bit although after a while it didn't seem to make much difference but initially it did, this was back in the early days. I tried medicinal mushrooms which were like a herbal medicine that an iridologist recommended to me. They made no difference although she told me some interesting facts about my family history, which were true, that was very impressive.

JD: (laughs) So the glucosamine did nothing for you?

AP: It might have done a bit but I didn't notice it.

JD: Some people recommend glucosamine for fatigue. It's interesting you say it didn't really work.

AP: Maybe I didn't try it for long enough.

JD: Did you try Saint John's Wort?

AP: No I never tried that! But I've been trying a number of vitamins for years, which I still do take because I'm sure they help in some way.

JD: Did you try anything other than supplements and vitamins?

AP: Yes reflexology! Nothing showed up there! EFT as well!

JD: Emotional Freedom Technique?

AP: Yes. I didn't fully pursue that, I should have had a few more sessions. I believe in all the holistic therapies but I just think that different ones work for different people and you've got to find the one that works for you.

JD: So what was it that finally worked for you?

AP: A couple of years ago I was just completely low on energy, this was after I'd been to the hospital and was told there was nothing wrong with me. So I thought I'd just try out a few random holistic therapies. Finally I saw a colonic hydrotherapist and she told me straight away that I was severely dehydrated and quite ill. I couldn't even have any treatments until I came back in a more hydrated state.

JD: Why do you think the doctor never picked up on dehydration?

AP: Because he never asked, he never probed enough. Even though he knew about my career as a dancer, they just put it down to, well you dance a lot and you just need to rest. But I knew that even when I'd rest for two or three weeks then I'd feel no different. I knew that it wasn't to do with the dance and there were others that did a lot more dancing than me and had worse diets and had lots more energy than I had.

JD: Explain what you did to rehydrate.

AP: I followed the instruction of the colonic hydrotherapist. She gave me a couple of other dietary things to look into. I can't actually remember what they were to be honest, but the main thing was she advised me to sip water all day every day. Warm water, cold water, any kind of water and go for two litres a day. My thirst instincts had completely shut down which meant that I struggled to drink the water at first. Because up until that point I'd only really been drinking three cups of tea a day.

JD: Were you never drinking water on its own at that point?

AP: I never drank water on its own!

JD: Even though you were a professional dancer?

AP: (laughs) I did occasionally have water but really not very often.

JD: What else were you drinking?

AP: Mainly just tea and coffee, I've never really been into fizzy drinks and I've never really drunk alcohol. Like I say, in general I've been really healthy. I've never smoked or drank alcohol and I've always had a good, healthy diet.

JD: So lots of sips of water all through the day is what you did?

AP: Gradually! At first my body couldn't take it. But I persisted with it and at first I was just fazed by one small bottle of water, which was a lot to take in. Maybe I could throughout the whole day, but certainly not within a couple of hours. I just couldn't manage it because my body was just not used to taking fluids. Then it was like my body realised that these fluids are trying to help me and then gradually I started to get really thirsty and it got to the point where I just drank and drank and drank and no matter how much I drank I just couldn't get rid of the thirst. I just thought this is crazy, how much do I need to drink to actually get rid of this thirst. I kept pursuing it and it was over a gradual, say two to three years to finally feel what I would actually class as normal, like everybody else.

JD: Two to three years is quite a long time. Did you gradually begin to feel better sooner than that?

AP: Yes! I'd began to feel better straight away, but over the years I had more and more energy and I was a lot more alert than I've ever been in my life. I feel sharp now and I don't feel groggy in the morning. Now I do tend to get more normal symptoms, like if I get a bit dehydrated I get a bit of a headache, I'd never ever had a headache before.

JD: How do you feel these days? Are you completely over your fatigue?

AP: I still feel like I'm thirsty from time to time. But my body tells me now, whereas before it never did. I never used to get symptoms of thirst, where my body tells me that I'm dehydrated, but now my body has taken the water and it knows when it needs more.

JD: How much better do you feel now compared to three years ago?

AP: I feel I've got at least double the energy, no at least triple (laughs). It's hard to put it into words because it's such a gradual thing, but I have at least triple the energy!

JD: And the only lifestyle change you made was to drink more water?

AP: Yes!

JD: Tell us more about your water (laughs).

AP: I buy bottled water and I drink tap water. Any water will do. I do prefer the taste of bottled water. Herbal teas as well! Herbal teas don't have caffeine in them, like the flower teas etc, I have them in the morning. The iridologist actually recommended nettle tea! That took me a while to get into it but now I actually enjoy it.

JD: Anything else you'd like to mention?

AP: Yes, I forgot to mention I was intolerant to dairy.

JD: Tell me what you want to say!

AP: Yes, the Iridologist told me I was allergic to dairy, this was before I saw the colonic hydrotherapist. This was before I knew I was dehydrated! I was told I was allergic to dairy and I would be all my life. So I cut dairy out.

JD: Were you taking in a lot of dairy before this?

AP: Yes! I used to over indulge in dairy without realising it. Dairy is in everything, if you have some crisps then you're having dairy!

JD: And now you drink oat milk? (my cup of tea had oat milk in it)

AP: (laughs) Well since the water, I've been able to gradually introduce dairy back and now I have absolutely no problem with dairy at all! That's just from drinking lots of water! But I do make sure I don't overindulge in dairy.

JD: And the doctor completely missed out on your dairy intolerance?

AP: The doctor missed out on everything. It was the Iridologist that found everything, they look into your eye, which is linked to your entire nervous system.

JD: That's about it for me, anything else you'd like to add?

AP: Just don't underestimate the power of water! It's made my skin improve and the quality of my hair too! It feels a lot softer now!

JD: How was your vision throughout all this, was it blurred?

AP: No, I've never had blurred vision, just blurred thinking.

JD: You still have that though!

AP: (laughs)

JD: Thanks!

Andrea Parker is a professional breakdance performer and instructor based in the north of England.

http://www.fireflyassociates.co.uk/

Printed in Great Britain
by Amazon.co.uk, Ltd.,
Marston Gate.